Competency-Based Logbook in
OBSTETRICS AND GYNECOLOGY
for MBBS

LOGBOOK

Name: _____

Roll No.: _____ Year: _____

College Name and Address: _____
_____
_____
_____

Competency-Based Logbook in
OBSTETRICS AND GYNECOLOGY for MBBS

As per the Competency-Based Medical Education Curriculum (NMC)

Arun Gupta

MS (Obstetrics and Gynecology)
Head and Senior Professor
Department of Obstetrics and Gynecology
Geetanjali Medical College and Hospital
Udaipur, Rajasthan, India

Neeraj R Mahajan

MD DNB (Physiology)
Associate Professor
Department of Physiology
Smt. NHL Municipal Medical College
Ahmedabad, Gujarat, India

Shabdika Kulshreshtha

MS (Obstetrics and Gynecology)
Associate Professor
Department of Obstetrics and Gynecology
Geetanjali Medical College and Hospital
Udaipur, Rajasthan, India

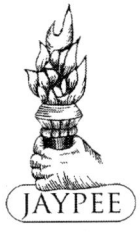

JAYPEE BROTHERS MEDICAL PUBLISHERS
The Health Sciences Publisher
New Delhi | London

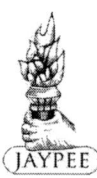

Jaypee Brothers Medical Publishers (P) Ltd.

Headquarters
Jaypee Brothers Medical Publishers (P) Ltd
EMCA House
23/23-B, Ansari Road, Daryaganj
New Delhi - 110 002, India
Landline: +91-11-23272143, +91-11-23272703
+91-11-23282021, +91-11-23245672
Email: jaypee@jaypeebrothers.com

Corporate Office
Jaypee Brothers Medical Publishers (P) Ltd
4838/24, Ansari Road, Daryaganj
New Delhi 110 002, India
Phone: +91-11-43574357
Fax: +91-11-43574314
Email: jaypee@jaypeebrothers.com

Overseas Office
J.P. Medical Ltd
83 Victoria Street, London
SW1H 0HW (UK)
Phone: +44 20 3170 8910
Fax: +44 (0)20 3008 6180
Email: info@jpmedpub.com

Website: www.jaypeebrothers.com
Website: www.jaypeedigital.com

© 2022, Jaypee Brothers Medical Publishers

The views and opinions expressed in this book are solely those of the original contributor(s)/author(s) and do not necessarily represent those of editor(s) and publisher of the book.

All rights reserved. No part of this publication may be reproduced, stored or transmitted in any form or by any means, electronic, mechanical, photocopying, recording or otherwise, without the prior permission in writing of the publishers.

All brand names and product names used in this book are trade names, service marks, trademarks or registered trademarks of their respective owners. The publisher is not associated with any product or vendor mentioned in this book.

Medical knowledge and practice change constantly. This book is designed to provide accurate, authoritative information about the subject matter in question. However, readers are advised to check the most current information available on procedures included and check information from the manufacturer of each product to be administered, to verify the recommended dose, formula, method and duration of administration, adverse effects and contraindications. It is the responsibility of the practitioner to take all appropriate safety precautions. Neither the publisher nor the author(s)/editor(s) assume any liability for any injury and/or damage to persons or property arising from or related to use of material in this book.

This book is sold on the understanding that the publisher is not engaged in providing professional medical services. If such advice or services are required, the services of a competent medical professional should be sought.

Every effort has been made where necessary to contact holders of copyright to obtain permission to reproduce copyright material. If any have been inadvertently overlooked, the publisher will be pleased to make the necessary arrangements at the first opportunity.

Inquiries for bulk sales may be solicited at: jaypee@jaypeebrothers.com

Competency-Based Logbook for Obstetrics and Gynecology for MBBS

First Edition: **2022,** Reprint: 2024

ISBN: 978-93-5465-766-5

Printed in India

Preface

Competency-Based Logbook for Obstetrics and Gynecology for MBBS is a verified and attested record of student's academic/cocurricular learning activities including all the three domains of knowledge, skills, ethics and communication. It strictly adheres to the performance level (P) competencies provided by the new NMC CBME curriculum in the subject of Obstetrics and Gynecology.

With the latest NMC guidelines, it is now mandatory for each student to maintain a logbook for each subject in MBBS. The subject of Obstetrics and Gynecology begins in phase 2 of MBBS so it becomes cumbersome to track the student's performance until phase 4 when the summative assessment takes place. So this logbook is prepared in such a manner that it reliably records the student's learning curve for a long duration of three and a half years.

This logbook is divided into various chapters based on the tools used to learn the clinical skills via clinical postings, skill laboratory, bedside clinics, DOAP sessions, small group discussions attended, self-directed learning (SDL) sessions, attitude, ethics and communication skills (AETCOM).

Few chapters are also dedicated to electives, pandemic module and seminar presentation.

Last chapter is dedicated to assessment record, reflective writing checklist, portfolio and certifiable competency (as per CBME).

As there is a single certifiable competency (as per new NMC CBME curriculum), so other competencies are also included which can be certified by the respective departments of the institute.

Arun Gupta
Neeraj R Mahajan
Shabdika Kulshreshtha

Student Profile

Name of Student: _____

Date of Joining: _____

Date of Birth: _____

Student's Contact No.: _____

Student's E-mail ID: _____

Parents Details

Father's Name: _____

Mobile No.: _____

Occupation: _____

Mother's Name: _____

Mobile No.: _____

Occupation: _____

Present Address: _____

_____

_____

Permanent Address: _____

_____

_____

Signature of Student

Certificate

This is to certify that this logbook is the bonafide work of Mr/Ms _____

Roll No. _____ Batch _____ in College _____

_____

_____

has successfully completed/has not completed all the skills/requirements mentioned in this logbook.

Further, it is certified that all the contents and entries made in logbook are true to the best of my knowledge.

Signature of HOD

Date:

General Instructions

- The logbook is a record of the academic/cocurricular activities of the designated student, who would be responsible for maintaining his/her logbook.
- The student is responsible for getting the entries in the logbook verified by the faculty in-charge regularly.
- Entries in the logbook will reflect the activities undertaken in the department and have to be scrutinized by the Head of the concerned department.
- The logbook is a record of various activities by the student like:
  - Overall participation and performance
  - Attendance
  - Participation in sessions
  - Record of completion of predetermined activities
  - Acquisition of selected competencies
- The logbook is the record of work done by the candidate in the department and will be verified by the college before submitting the application of the students for the university examination.
- As per the CBME, reflection writing is an important teaching learning method as well as an assessment tool, so this logbook contains the structured guidelines/checklist for reflection writing.
- **OG 13.5, i.e., observing and assisting normal delivery is the only certifiable competency in the subject as per NMC, so other certifiable competencies are also suggested phase wise which can be included in the logbook. A flexible approach can be adopted by the faculties in the respective Obstetrics and Gynecology departments of the Institute.**

Contents

1. Clinical Posting — 1
   - Phase-wise Classification of All Psychomotor Competencies *1*
2. Skill Laboratory — 8
3. Bedside Clinics — 9
4. Demonstrate, Observe, Assist, Perform (DOAP) Sessions — 12
5. Small Group Discussions Attended — 15
6. Self-directed Learning (SDL) Sessions — 17
   - First Contact Session *17*
   - Second Contact Session *17*
7. Attitude, Ethics and Communication (AETCOM) Competencies — 27
8. Electives-Block-2 — 29
   - Reflection Writing *30*
9. Pandemic Module — 39
10. Seminar Presented — 40
11. Scientific Contribution — 41
    - Record of Assessment *41*
    - Checklist for Reflective Writing *42*
    - Reflective Writing is based on Gibbs and Kolb's Reflective Learning Cycle (AAAA) *42*
    - Reflective Writing *43*
    - Portfolio (Part A) *47*
    - Certifiable Competency (As per CBME) *50*
    - Other Certifiable Competencies *51*

CLINICAL POSTING

Phase	Semester	From (date)	To (date)	Unit	Concerned faculty
II					
III Part 1					
IV Part 2					

■ PHASE-WISE CLASSIFICATION OF ALL PSYCHOMOTOR COMPETENCIES

IInd Year MBBS

Number of competency addressed	Name of activity	Date completed dd-mm-yyyy	Attempt at activity First or Only (F) Repeat (R) Remedial (Re)	Rating Below (B) expectations Meets (M) expectations Exceeds (E) expectations	Decision of faculty Completed (C) Repeat (R) Remedial (Re)	Initial of faculty and date	Feedback received Initial of learner
Topic: Diagnosis of pregnancy							
OG6.1	Describe, discuss and demonstrate the clinical features of pregnancy, derive and discuss its differential diagnosis, elaborate the principles underlying and interpret pregnancy tests.						
Topic: Antenatal care							
OG8.2	Elicit document and present an obstetric history including menstrual history, last menstrual period, previous obstetric history, comorbid conditions, past medical history and surgical history.						
OG8.3	Describe, demonstrate, document and perform an obstetrical examination including a general and abdominal examination and clinical monitoring of maternal and fetal well-being.						

Number of competency addressed	Name of activity	Date completed dd-mm-yyyy	Attempt at activity First or Only (F) Repeat (R) Remedial (Re)	Rating Below (B) expectations Meets (M) expectations Exceeds (E) expectations	Decision of faculty Completed (C) Repeat (R) Remedial (Re)	Initial of faculty and date	Feedback received Initial of learner
OG8.4	Describe and demonstrate clinical monitoring of maternal and fetal well-being.						
OG8.5	Describe and demonstrate pelvic assessment in a model.						
OG8.6	Assess and counsel a patient in a simulated environment regarding appropriate nutrition in pregnancy.						
OG17.2	Counsel in a simulated environment, care of the breast, importance and the technique of breastfeeding.						
OG18.2	Demonstrate the steps of neonatal resuscitation in a simulated environment.						
OG20.2	In a simulated environment administer informed consent to a person wishing to undergo medical termination of pregnancy (MTP).						
OG35.1	Obtain a logical sequence of history, and perform a humane and thorough clinical examination, excluding internal examinations (per-rectal and per-vaginal).						
OG35.3	Recognize situations, which call for urgent or early treatment at secondary and tertiary centers and make a prompt referral of such patients after giving first aid or emergency treatment.						
OG35.4	Demonstrate interpersonal and communication skills befitting a physician in order to discuss illness and its outcome with patient and family.						
OG35.5	Determine gestational age, EDD and obstetric formula.						
OG35.6	Demonstrate ethical behavior in all aspects of medical practice.						
OG35.7	Obtain informed consent for any examination/procedure.						

Number of competency addressed	Name of activity	Date completed dd-mm-yyyy	Attempt at activity First or Only (F) Repeat (R) Remedial (Re)	Rating Below (B) expectations Meets (M) expectations Exceeds (E) expectations	Decision of faculty Completed (C) Repeat (R) Remedial (Re)	Initial of faculty and date	Feedback received Initial of learner
OG35.11	Demonstrate the correct use of appropriate universal precautions for self-protection against HIV and hepatitis and counsel patients.						
AN49.1	Describe and demonstrate the superficial and deep perineal pouch (boundaries and contents).						
AN49.2	Describe and identify perineal body.						
AN53.1	Identify and hold the bone in the anatomical position, Describe the salient features, articulations and demonstrate the attachments of muscle groups.						
AN53.2	Demonstrate anatomical position of bony pelvis and show boundaries of pelvic inlet, pelvic cavity, pelvic outlet.						
AN53.3	Define true pelvis and false pelvis and demonstrate sex determination in male and female bony pelvis.						
AN64.3	Describe various types of open neural tube defects with its embryological basis.						
PA22.2	Enumerate the indications describe the principles enumerate and demonstrate the steps of compatibility testing.						
PE18.5	Provide intranatal care and observe the conduct of a normal delivery.						
Topic: Complications in early pregnancy							
OG9.2	Describe the steps and observe/assist in the performance of an MTP evacuation.						

IIIrd Year MBBS

Number of competency addressed	Name of activity	Date completed dd-mm-yyyy	Attempt at activity First or Only (F) Repeat (R) Remedial (Re)	Rating Below (B) expectations Meets (M) expectations Exceeds (E) expectations	Decision of faculty Completed (C) Repeat (R) Remedial (Re)	Initial of faculty and date	Feedback received Initial of learner
Topic: Diagnosis of pregnancy							
OG13.3	Observe/assist in the performance of an artificial rupture of membranes.						
OG13.4	Demonstrate the stages of normal labor in a simulated environment/mannequin and counsel on methods of safe abortion.						
OG13.5	Observe and assist the conduct of a normal vaginal delivery.						
OG19.2	Counsel in a simulated environment, contraception and puerperal sterilization.						
OG19.3	Observe/assist in the performance of tubal ligation.						
OG19.4	Enumerate the indications for, describe the steps in and insert and remove an intrauterine device in a simulated environment.						
OG31.1	Describe and discuss the etiology, classification, clinical features, diagnosis, investigations, principles of management and preventive aspects of prolapse of uterus.						
Topic: Obstetrics and gynecological skills - I		**Number of competencies: (05)**					
OG35.2	Arrive at a logical provisional diagnosis after examination.						
OG35.8	Write a complete case record with all necessary details.						
OG35.13	Demonstrate the correct technique to perform artificial rupture of membranes in a simulated/supervised environment.						
OG35.16	Diagnose and provide emergency management of antepartum and postpartum hemorrhage in a simulated/guided environment.						
OG35.17	Demonstrate the correct technique of urinary catheterization in a simulated/supervised environment.						

IVth Year MBBS

Number of competency addressed	Name of activity	Date completed dd-mm-yyyy	Attempt at activity First or Only (F) Repeat (R) Remedial (Re)	Rating Below (B) expectations Meets (M) expectations Exceeds (E) expectations	Decision of faculty Completed (C) Repeat (R) Remedial (Re)	Initial of faculty and date	Feedback received Initial of learner
Topic: Preconception counseling							
OG5.1	Describe, discuss and identify pre-existing medical disorders and discuss their management; discuss evidence-based intrapartum care.						
OG5.2	Determine maternal high risk factors and verify immunization status.						
OG13.3	Observe/assist in the performance of an artificial rupture of membranes.						
OG13.4	Demonstrate the stages of normal labor in a simulated environment/mannequin and counsel on methods of safe abortion.						
OG13.5	Observe and assist the conduct of a normal vaginal delivery.						
OG15.2	Observe and assist in the performance of an episiotomy and demonstrate the correct suturing technique of an episiotomy in a simulated environment. Observe/assist in operative obstetrics cases—including: CS, forceps, vacuum extraction, and breech delivery.						
OG35.10	Write a proper referral note to secondary or tertiary centers or to other physicians with all necessary details.						
OG35.15	Demonstrate the correct technique to insert and remove an IUD in a simulated/supervised environment.						

Number of competency addressed	Name of activity	Date completed dd-mm-yyyy	Attempt at activity First or Only (F) Repeat (R) Remedial (Re)	Rating Below (B) expectations Meets (M) expectations Exceeds (E) expectations	Decision of faculty Completed (C) Repeat (R) Remedial (Re)	Initial of faculty and date	Feedback received Initial of learner
OG35.17	Demonstrate the correct technique of urinary catheterization in a simulated/supervised environment.						
OG33.3	Describe and demonstrate the screening for cervical cancer in a simulated environment.						
OG34.4	Operative Gynecology: Understand and describe the technique and complications: Dilatation and Curettage (D and C); EA-ECC; cervical biopsy; abdominal hysterectomy; myomectomy; surgery for ovarian tumours; staging laparotomy; vaginal hysterectomy including pelvic floor repair; Fothergill's operation, Laparoscopy; hysteroscopy; management of postoperative complications.						
OG36.1	Plan and institute a line of treatment, which is need based, cost effective and appropriate for common conditions taking into consideration: • Patient • Disease • Socioeconomic status • Institution/Governmental guidelines.						
OG36.3	Demonstrate the correct technique of punch biopsy of uterus in a simulated/supervised environment.						
OG37.1	Observe and assist in the performance of a cesarean section.						
OG37.2	Observe and assist in the performance of laparotomy.						

Number of competency addressed	Name of activity	Date completed dd-mm-yyyy	Attempt at activity First or Only (F) Repeat (R) Remedial (Re)	Rating Below (B) expectations Meets (M) expectations Exceeds (E) expectations	Decision of faculty Completed (C) Repeat (R) Remedial (Re)	Initial of faculty and date	Feedback received Initial of learner
OG37.3	Observe and assist in the performance of Hysterectomy – abdominal/vaginal.						
OG37.4	Observe and assist in the performance of dilatation and curettage (D and C).						
OG37.5	Observe and assist in the performance of endometrial aspiration-endocervical curettage (EA-ECC).						
OG37.6	Observe and assist in the performance of outlet forceps application of vacuum and breech delivery.						
OG37.7	Observe and assist in the performance of MTP in the first trimester and evacuation in incomplete abortion.						
OG35.9	Write a proper discharge summary with all relevant information.						
OG35.12	Obtain a PAP smear in a stimulated environment.						
OG35.14	Demonstrate the correct technique to perform and suture episiotomies in a simulated/supervised environment.						

SKILL LABORATORY

	IInd year MBBS						
	As per the competencies given by NMC No Class to be taken in skill laboratory in this phase						
	IIIrd year MBBS						
PE7.7	Perform breast examination and identify common problems during lactation such as retracted nipples, cracked nipples, breast engorgement, breast abscess.						
PE18.5	Provide intranatal care and conduct a normal delivery in a simulated environment.						
PE18.6	Perform postnatal assessment of newborn and mother, provide advice on breastfeeding, weaning and on family planning.						
	IVth year MBBS						
PE32.6	Interpret normal karyotype and recognize the Turner karyotype.						
OG34.4	Operative gynecology: Understand and describe the technique and complications: Dilatation and curettage (D and C); EA-ECC; cervical biopsy; abdominal hysterectomy; myomectomy; surgery for ovarian tumors; staging laparotomy; vaginal hysterectomy including pelvic floor repair; Fothergill's operation, laparoscopy; hysteroscopy; management of postoperative complications.						

BEDSIDE CLINICS

Number of competency addressed	Name of activity	Date completed dd-mm-yyyy	Attempt at activity First or Only (F) Repeat (R) Remedial (Re)	Rating Below (B) expectations Meets (M) expectations Exceeds (E) expectations	Decision of faculty Completed (C) Repeat (R) Remedial (Re)	Initial of faculty and date	Feedback received Initial of learner
		IInd year MBBS					
OG6.1	Describe, discuss and demonstrate the clinical features of pregnancy, derive and discuss its differential diagnosis, elaborate the principles underlying and interpret pregnancy tests.						
OG8.2	Elicit document and present an obstetric history including menstrual history, last menstrual period, previous obstetric history, comorbid conditions, past medical history and surgical history.						
OG8.3	• Describe, demonstrate, document and perform an obstetrical examination including a general and abdominal examination and clinical monitoring of maternal and fetal well-being.						
	• Describe and demonstrate clinical monitoring of maternal and fetal well-being.						
OG8.6	Assess and counsel a patient in a simulated environment regarding appropriate nutrition in pregnancy.						
OG35.1	Obtain a logical sequence of history, and perform a humane and thorough clinical examination, excluding internal examinations (per-rectal and per-vaginal).						
OG35.3	Recognize situations, which call for urgent or early treatment at secondary and tertiary centers and make a prompt referral of such patients after giving first aid or emergency treatment.						
OG35.4	Demonstrate interpersonal and communication skills befitting a physician in order to discuss illness and its outcome with patient and family.						
OG35.5	Determine gestational age, EDD and obstetric formula.						

Number of competency addressed	Name of activity	Date completed dd-mm-yyyy	Attempt at activity First or Only (F) Repeat (R) Remedial (Re)	Rating Below (B) expectations Meets (M) expectations Exceeds (E) expectations	Decision of faculty Completed (C) Repeat (R) Remedial (Re)	Initial of faculty and date	Feedback received Initial of learner
OG35.6	Demonstrate ethical behavior in all aspects of medical practice.						
OG35.7	Obtain informed consent for any examination/procedure.						
IIIrd year MBBS							
OG9.2	Describe the steps and observe/assist in the performance of an MTP evacuation.						
OG13.3	Observe/assist in the performance of an artificial rupture of membranes.						
OG35.2	Arrive at a logical provisional diagnosis after examination.						
OG5.8	Write a complete case record with all necessary details.						
PE7.7	Perform breast examination and identify common problems during lactation such as retracted nipples, cracked nipples, breast engorgement, breast abscess.						
PE18.3	Conduct antenatal examination of women independently and apply at-risk approach in antenatal care						
PE18.6	Perform postnatal assessment of newborn and mother, provide advice on breastfeeding, weaning and on family planning.						
IVth year MBBS							
	Describe, discuss and identify pre-existing medical disorders and discuss their management; discuss evidence-based intrapartum care.						
	Determine maternal high risk factors and verify immunization status.						
OG15.2	Observe and assist in the performance of an episiotomy and demonstrate the correct suturing technique of an episiotomy in a simulated environment. Observe/assist in operative obstetrics cases—including: CS, forceps, vacuum extraction, and breech delivery.						

Number of competency addressed	Name of activity	Date completed dd-mm-yyyy	Attempt at activity First or Only (F) Repeat (R) Remedial (Re)	Rating Below (B) expectations Meets (M) expectations Exceeds (E) expectations	Decision of faculty Completed (C) Repeat (R) Remedial (Re)	Initial of faculty and date	Feedback received Initial of learner
OG35.10	Write a proper referral note to secondary or tertiary centers or to other physicians with all necessary details.						
OG36.1	Plan and institute a line of treatment, which is need based, cost effective and appropriate for common conditions taking into consideration: • Patient • Disease • Socioeconomic status • Institution/Governmental guidelines.						
OG36.3	Demonstrate the correct technique of punch biopsy of uterus in a simulated/supervised environment.						
OG37.1	Observe and assist in the performance of a cesarean section.						
OG37.2	Observe and assist in the performance of laparotomy.						
OG37.3	Observe and assist in the performance of hysterectomy—abdominal/vaginal.						
OG37.4	Observe and assist in the performance of dilatation and curettage (D and C).						
OG37.5	Observe and assist in the performance of endometrial aspiration-endocervical curettage (EA-ECC).						
OG37.6	Observe and assist in the performance of outlet forceps application of vacuum and breech delivery.						
OG37.7	Observe and assist in the performance of MTP in the first trimester and evacuation in incomplete abortion.						
PE32.8	Interpret normal karyotype and recognize the Turner karyotype.						

DEMONSTRATE, OBSERVE, ASSIST, PERFORM (DOAP) SESSIONS

Number of competency addressed	Name of activity	Date completed dd-mm-yyyy	Attempt at activity First or Only (F) Repeat (R) Remedial (Re)	Rating Below (B) expectations Meets (M) expectations Exceeds (E) expectations	Decision of faculty Completed (C) Repeat (R) Remedial (Re)	Initial of faculty and date	Feedback received Initial of learner
			IInd year MBBS				
OG8.3	Describe, demonstrate, document and perform an obstetrical examination including a general and abdominal examination and clinical monitoring of maternal and fetal well-being.						
OG8.4	Describe and demonstrate clinical monitoring of maternal and fetal well-being.						
OG8.4	Describe and demonstrate pelvic assessment in a model.						
OG8.5	Assess and counsel a patient in a simulated environment regarding appropriate nutrition in pregnancy.						
OG17.2	Counsel in a simulated environment, care of the breast, importance and the technique of breastfeeding.						
OG18.2	Demonstrate the steps of neonatal resuscitation in a simulated environment.						
OG20.2	In a simulated environment administer informed consent to a person wishing to undergo medical termination of pregnancy (MTP).						
OG35.11	Demonstrate the correct use of appropriate universal precautions for self-protection against HIV and hepatitis and counsel patients.						
AN49.1	Describe and demonstrate the superficial and deep perineal pouch (boundaries and contents).						
AN49.2	Describe and identify perineal body.						
AN53.1	Identify and hold the bone in the anatomical position, describe the salient features, articulations and demonstrate the attachments of muscle groups.						

Number of competency addressed	Name of activity	Date completed dd-mm-yyyy	Attempt at activity First or Only (F) Repeat (R) Remedial (Re)	Rating Below (B) expectations Meets (M) expectations Exceeds (E) expectations	Decision of faculty Completed (C) Repeat (R) Remedial (Re)	Initial of faculty and date	Feedback received Initial of learner
AN53.2	Demonstrate anatomical position of bony pelvis and show boundaries of pelvic inlet, pelvic cavity, pelvic outlet.						
AN53.3	Define true pelvis and false pelvis and demonstrate sex determination in male and female bony pelvis.						
IIIrd year MBBS							
OG9.2	Describe the steps and observe/assist in the performance of an MTP evacuation.						
OG13.3	• Observe/assist in the performance of an artificial rupture of membranes.						
	• Demonstrate the stages of normal labor in a simulated environment/mannequin and counsel on methods of safe abortion.						
OG13.5	• Observe and assist the conduct of a normal vaginal delivery.						
	• Counsel in a simulated environment, contraception and puerperal sterilization.						
OG19.3	Observe/assist in the performance of tubal ligation.						
OG19.4	Enumerate the indications for, describe the steps in and insert and remove an intrauterine device in a simulated environment.						
OG35.13	Demonstrate the correct technique to perform artificial rupture of membranes in a simulated/supervised environment.						
OG35.14	Demonstrate the correct technique to perform and suture episiotomies in a simulated/supervised environment.						
OG35.16	Diagnose and provide emergency management of antepartum and postpartum hemorrhage in a simulated/guided environment.						
OG35.17	Demonstrate the correct technique of urinary catheterization in a simulated/supervised environment.						

Number of competency addressed	Name of activity	Date completed dd-mm-yyyy	Attempt at activity First or Only (F) Repeat (R) Remedial (Re)	Rating Below (B) expectations Meets (M) expectations Exceeds (E) expectations	Decision of faculty Completed (C) Repeat (R) Remedial (Re)	Initial of faculty and date	Feedback received Initial of learner
CM9.2	Define, calculate and interpret demographic indices including birth rate, death rate, fertility rates.						
PE7.8	Educate mothers on antenatal breast care and prepare mothers for lactation.						
PE7.0	Educate and counsel mothers for best practices in breastfeeding.						
PE18.5	Provide intranatal care and conduct a normal delivery in a simulated environment.						
IVth year MBBS							
OG13.3	Observe/assist in the performance of an artificial rupture of membranes.						
OG134	Demonstrate the stages of normal labor in a simulated environment/mannequin and counsel on methods of safe abortion.						
OG35.12	Obtain a PAP smear in a stimulated environment.						
OG13.5	Observe and assist the conduct of a normal vaginal delivery.						
OG15.2	Observe and assist in the performance of an episiotomy and demonstrate the correct suturing technique of an episiotomy in a simulated environment. Observe/assist in operative obstetrics cases— including: CS, forceps, vacuum extraction, and breech delivery.						
OG35.15	Demonstrate the correct technique to insert and remove an IUD in a simulated/supervised environment.						
OG35.17	Demonstrate the correct technique of urinary catheterization in a simulated/supervised environment.						
PE20.6	Explain the follow up care for neonates including breastfeeding, temperature maintenance, immunization, importance of growth monitoring and red flags.						

SMALL GROUP DISCUSSION ATTENDED

Number of competency addressed	Name of activity	Date completed dd-mm-yyyy	Attempt at activity First or Only (F) Repeat (R) Remedial (Re)	Rating Below (B) expectations Meets (M) expectations Exceeds (E) expectations	Decision of faculty Completed (C) Repeat (R) Remedial (Re)	Initial of faculty and date	Feedback received Initial of learner
			IInd year MBBS				
OG6.1	Describe, discuss and demonstrate the clinical features of pregnancy, derive and discuss its differential diagnosis, elaborate the principles underlying and interpret pregnancy tests.						
OG8.2	Elicit document and present an obstetric history including menstrual history, last menstrual period, previous obstetric history, comorbid conditions, past medical history and surgical history.						
AN49.1	Describe and demonstrate the superficial and deep perineal pouch (boundaries and contents).						
AN49.2	Describe and identify perineal body.						
PA32.2	Enumerate the indications describe the principles enumerate and demonstrate the steps of compatibility testing.						
			IIIrd year MBBS				
OG9.2	Describe the steps and observe/assist in the performance of an MTP evacuation.						
PE18.6	Perform postnatal assessment of newborn and mother, provide advice on breastfeeding, weaning and on family planning.						
			IVth year MBBS				
OG36.1	Plan and institute a line of treatment, which is need based, cost effective and appropriate for common conditions taking into consideration: • Patient • Disease • Socioeconomic status • Institution/Governmental guidelines.						

Number of competency addressed	Name of activity	Date completed dd-mm-yyyy	Attempt at activity First or Only (F) Repeat (R) Remedial (Re)	Rating Below (B) expectations Meets (M) expectations Exceeds (E) expectations	Decision of faculty Completed (C) Repeat (R) Remedial (Re)	Initial of faculty and date	Feedback received Initial of learner
OG37.1	Observe and assist in the performance of a cesarean section.						
OG37.2	Observe and assist in the performance of laparotomy.						
OG37.3	Observe and assist in the performance of hysterectomy—abdominal/vaginal.						
OG37.4	Observe and assist in the performance of dilatation and curettage (D and C).						
OG37.5	Observe and assist in the performance of endometrial aspiration-endocervical curettage (EA-ECC).						
OG37.6	Observe and assist in the performance of outlet forceps application of vacuum and breech delivery.						
OG37.7	Observe and assist in the performance of MTP in the first trimester and evacuation in incomplete abortion.						

SELF-DIRECTED LEARNING (SDL) SESSIONS

Topic: _____   Date: _____

■ FIRST CONTACT SESSION

1. Learning objectives: _____
   _____
   _____

2. Suggested resource material: _____
   _____
   _____

3. Milestones (time line): _____
   _____

Intersession Period Duration

■ SECOND CONTACT SESSION

1. Output: _____
2. Answers: _____
3. Grading by faculty: _____
4. Self/peer assessment: _____
5. Feedback: _____
6. Reflection: _____

Faculty Name: _____

Sign/Seal: _____

Date: _____

SELF-DIRECTED LEARNING (SDL) SESSIONS

Topic: _____   Date: _____

■ FIRST CONTACT SESSION

1. Learning objectives: _____
   _____
   _____

2. Suggested resource material: _____
   _____
   _____

3. Milestones (time line): _____
   _____
   _____

Intersession Period Duration

■ SECOND CONTACT SESSION

1. Output: _____
   _____
2. Answers: _____
   _____
3. Grading by faculty: _____
   _____
4. Self/peer assessment: _____
   _____
5. Feedback: _____
   _____
6. Reflection: _____
   _____

Faculty Name: _____

Sign/Seal: _____

Date: _____

SELF-DIRECTED LEARNING (SDL) SESSIONS

Topic: _____   Date: _____

■ FIRST CONTACT SESSION

1. Learning objectives: _____
   _____
   _____

2. Suggested resource material: _____
   _____
   _____

3. Milestones (time line): _____
   _____
   _____

Intersession Period Duration

■ SECOND CONTACT SESSION

1. Output: _____
   _____

2. Answers: _____
   _____

3. Grading by faculty: _____
   _____

4. Self/peer assessment: _____
   _____

5. Feedback: _____
   _____

6. Reflection: _____
   _____

Faculty Name: _____

Sign/Seal: _____

Date: _____

SELF-DIRECTED LEARNING (SDL) SESSIONS

Topic: _____ Date: _____

■ FIRST CONTACT SESSION

1. Learning objectives: _____
   _____
   _____

2. Suggested resource material: _____
   _____
   _____

3. Milestones (time line): _____
   _____
   _____

Intersession Period Duration

■ SECOND CONTACT SESSION

1. Output: _____
   _____

2. Answers: _____
   _____

3. Grading by faculty: _____
   _____

4. Self/peer assessment: _____
   _____

5. Feedback: _____
   _____

6. Reflection: _____
   _____

Faculty Name: _____

Sign/Seal: _____

Date: _____

SELF-DIRECTED LEARNING (SDL) SESSIONS

Topic: _____   Date: _____

FIRST CONTACT SESSION

1. Learning objectives: _____
   _____
   _____

2. Suggested resource material: _____
   _____
   _____

3. Milestones (time line): _____
   _____
   _____

Intersession Period Duration

SECOND CONTACT SESSION

1. Output: _____
   _____

2. Answers: _____
   _____

3. Grading by faculty: _____
   _____

4. Self/peer assessment: _____
   _____

5. Feedback: _____
   _____

6. Reflection: _____
   _____

Faculty Name: _____

Sign/Seal: _____

Date: _____

SELF-DIRECTED LEARNING (SDL) SESSIONS

Topic: _____   Date: _____

FIRST CONTACT SESSION

1. Learning objectives: _____
   _____
   _____

2. Suggested resource material: _____
   _____
   _____

3. Milestones (time line): _____
   _____
   _____

Intersession Period Duration

SECOND CONTACT SESSION

1. Output: _____
   _____

2. Answers: _____

3. Grading by faculty: _____

4. Self/peer assessment: _____

5. Feedback: _____

6. Reflection: _____
   _____

Faculty Name: _____

Sign/Seal: _____

Date: _____

SELF-DIRECTED LEARNING (SDL) SESSIONS

Topic: _____   Date: _____

■ FIRST CONTACT SESSION

1. Learning objectives: _____
   _____
   _____

2. Suggested resource material: _____
   _____
   _____

3. Milestones (time line): _____
   _____
   _____

Intersession Period Duration

■ SECOND CONTACT SESSION

1. Output: _____

2. Answers: _____

3. Grading by faculty: _____

4. Self/peer assessment: _____
   _____

5. Feedback: _____
   _____

6. Reflection: _____
   _____

Faculty Name: _____

Sign/Seal: _____

Date: _____

SELF-DIRECTED LEARNING (SDL) SESSIONS

Topic: _____   Date: _____

■ FIRST CONTACT SESSION

1. Learning objectives: _____
   _____
   _____

2. Suggested resource material: _____
   _____
   _____

3. Milestones (time line): _____
   _____
   _____

Intersession Period Duration

■ SECOND CONTACT SESSION

1. Output: _____
   _____

2. Answers: _____
   _____

3. Grading by faculty: _____
   _____

4. Self/peer assessment: _____
   _____

5. Feedback: _____
   _____

6. Reflection: _____
   _____

Faculty Name: _____

Sign/Seal: _____

Date: _____

SELF-DIRECTED LEARNING (SDL) SESSIONS

Topic: _____   Date: _____

■ FIRST CONTACT SESSION

1. Learning objectives: _____
   _____
   _____

2. Suggested resource material: _____
   _____
   _____

3. Milestones (time line): _____
   _____
   _____

Intersession Period Duration

■ SECOND CONTACT SESSION

1. Output: _____
2. Answers: _____
3. Grading by faculty: _____
4. Self/peer assessment: _____
5. Feedback: _____
6. Reflection: _____
   _____

Faculty Name: _____

Sign/Seal: _____

Date: _____

SELF-DIRECTED LEARNING (SDL) SESSIONS

Topic: _____ Date: _____

■ FIRST CONTACT SESSION

1. Learning objectives: _____
   _____
   _____

2. Suggested resource material: _____
   _____
   _____

3. Milestones (time line): _____
   _____
   _____

Intersession Period Duration

■ SECOND CONTACT SESSION

1. Output: _____
   _____

2. Answers: _____

3. Grading by faculty: _____

4. Self/peer assessment: _____

5. Feedback: _____

6. Reflection: _____
   _____

Faculty Name: _____

Sign/Seal: _____

Date: _____

ATTITUDE, ETHICS AND COMMUNICATION (AETCOM) COMPETENCIES

Number of competency addressed	Name of activity	Date completed dd-mm-yyyy	Attempt at activity First or Only (F) Repeat (R) Remedial (Re)	Rating Below (B) expectations Meets (M) expectations Exceeds (E) expectations	Decision of faculty Completed (C) Repeat (R) Remedial (Re)	Initial of faculty and date	Feedback received Initial of learner
			IInd year MBBS				
OG17.2	Counsel in a simulated environment, care of the breast, importance and the technique of breastfeeding.						
OG20.2	In a simulated environment administer informed consent to a person wishing to undergo medical termination of pregnancy (MTP).						
OG35.4	Demonstrate interpersonal and communication skills befitting a physician in order to discuss illness and its outcome with patient and family.						
OG35.6	Demonstrate ethical behavior in all aspects of medical practice.						
PE7.8	Educate mothers on antenatal breast care and prepare mothers for lactation.						
PE7.9	Educate and counsel mothers for best practices in breastfeeding.						
			IIIrd year MBBS				
OG19.2	Counsel in a simulated environment, contraception and puerperal sterilization.						
PE7.8	Educate mothers on antenatal breast care and prepare mothers for lactation.						
PE7.9	Educate and counsel mothers for best practices in breastfeeding.						
			IVth year MBBS				
OG37.1	Observe and assist in the performance of a cesarean section.						
OG37.2	Observe and assist in the performance of laparotomy.						
OG37.3	Observe and assist in the performance of hysterectomy—abdominal/vaginal.						
OG37.4	Observe and assist in the performance of dilatation and curettage (D and C).						

Number of competency addressed	Name of activity	Date completed dd-mm-yyyy	Attempt at activity First or Only (F) Repeat (R) Remedial (Re)	Rating Below (B) expectations Meets (M) expectations Exceeds (E) expectations	Decision of faculty Completed (C) Repeat (R) Remedial (Re)	Initial of faculty and date	Feedback received Initial of learner
OG37.5	Observe and assist in the performance of endometrial aspiration-endocervical curettage (EA-ECC).						
OG37.6	Observe and assist in the performance of outlet forceps application of vacuum and breech delivery.						
OG37.7	Observe and assist in the performance of MTP in the first trimester and evacuation in incomplete abortion.						

ELECTIVES-BLOCK-2

Name of the elective: _____
_____
_____
_____

Location of the hospital/research facility: _____
_____
_____
_____

Learning objectives of elective: _____
_____
_____
_____

Prerequisites of elective: _____
_____
_____
_____

List of activities of student participation: _____
_____
_____
_____

Learning resources: _____
_____
_____
_____

Remarks: _____
_____
_____
_____

Name of Internal Preceptor(s): _____

Sign: _____

Date: _____

Name of External Preceptor (If Applicable)

Sign: _____

Date: _____

REFLECTION WRITING

What Happened?

_____
_____
_____
_____
_____
_____
_____
_____

So What?

_____
_____
_____
_____
_____
_____
_____
_____

What's Next?

_____
_____
_____
_____
_____
_____
_____
_____

ELECTIVES-BLOCK-2

Name of the elective: _____
_____
_____
_____

Location of the hospital/research facility: _____
_____
_____
_____

Learning objectives of elective: _____
_____
_____
_____

Prerequisites of elective: _____
_____
_____
_____

List of activities of student participation: _____
_____
_____
_____

Learning resources: _____
_____
_____
_____

Remarks: _____
_____
_____

Name of Internal Preceptor(s): _____

Sign: _____

Date: _____

Name of External Preceptor (If Applicable)

Sign: _____

Date: _____

REFLECTION WRITING

What Happened?

_____

So What?

_____

What's Next?

_____

ELECTIVES-BLOCK-2

Name of the elective: _____
_____
_____
_____

Location of the hospital/research facility: _____
_____
_____
_____

Learning objectives of elective: _____
_____
_____
_____

Prerequisites of elective: _____
_____
_____
_____

List of activities of student participation: _____
_____
_____
_____

Learning resources: _____
_____
_____
_____

Remarks: _____
_____
_____
_____

Name of Internal Preceptor(s): _____

Sign: _____

Date: _____

Name of External Preceptor (If Applicable)

Sign: _____

Date: _____

REFLECTION WRITING

What Happened?

So What?

What's Next?

ELECTIVES-BLOCK-2

Name of the elective: _____
_____
_____
_____

Location of the hospital/research facility: _____
_____
_____
_____

Learning objectives of elective: _____
_____
_____
_____

Prerequisites of elective: _____
_____
_____
_____

List of activities of student participation: _____
_____
_____
_____

Learning resources: _____
_____
_____
_____

Remarks: _____
_____
_____
_____

Name of Internal Preceptor(s): _____

Sign: _____

Date: _____

Name of External Preceptor (If Applicable)

Sign: _____

Date: _____

REFLECTION WRITING

What Happened?

So What?

What's Next?

ELECTIVES-BLOCK-2

Name of the elective: _____
_____
_____
_____

Location of the hospital/research facility: _____
_____
_____
_____

Learning objectives of elective: _____
_____
_____
_____

Prerequisites of elective: _____
_____
_____
_____

List of activities of student participation: _____
_____
_____
_____

Learning resources: _____
_____
_____
_____

Remarks: _____
_____
_____
_____

Name of Internal Preceptor(s): _____

Sign: _____

Date: _____

Name of External Preceptor (If Applicable)

Sign: _____

Date: _____

REFLECTION WRITING

What Happened?

_____

So What?

_____

What's Next?

_____

PANDEMIC MODULE

Number of competency addressed	Name of activity	Date completed dd-mm-yyyy	Attempt at activity First or Only (F) Repeat (R) Remedial (Re)	Rating Below (B) expectations Meets (M) expectations Exceeds (E) expectations	Decision of faculty Completed (C) Repeat (R) Remedial (Re)	Initial of faculty and date	Feedback received Initial of learner

SEMINAR PRESENTED

Number of competency addressed	Name of activity	Date completed dd-mm-yyyy	Attempt at activity First or Only (F) Repeat (R) Remedial (Re)	Rating Below (B) expectations Meets (M) expectations Exceeds (E) expectations	Decision of faculty Completed (C) Repeat (R) Remedial (Re)	Initial of faculty and date	Feedback received Initial of learner

SCIENTIFIC CONTRIBUTION

Sl. No.	ICMR STS project	Remarks

Signature of Student **Signature of HOD**

RECORD OF ASSESSMENT

Assessment method	Max. marks	Min. marks	Marks obtained

Remarks:

Signature of HOD

Note: Above information is for the benefit of students and parents. In case of any discrepancy departmental record will be treated as final.

CHECKLIST FOR REFLECTIVE WRITING

What happened?
• What was the **session** and who **conducted** it?
So what?
• What **key points** did I take away from the sessions? • What **interested and motivated me** about these sessions? • What were **new skills and information** or understanding for me? • Describe **holistic learning** (skill, attitude, knowledge, communication, emotional, psychological, all) • **Why I learned** what I learned and **Why I can't learn** what I can't learned? • **How I learned best?** (learning style) • Include both **good and bad points** and why • Include both **professional and personal** gains
What next?
• **How will I** use this learning for the benefit of **society** and will this learning shape me up into a **better doctor**? Then what ideas I should use **immediately** and which ones, better for **future** application?

REFLECTIVE WRITING IS BASED ON GIBBS AND KOLB'S REFLECTIVE LEARNING CYCLE (AAAA)

Any experience
↓
Affect/feelings (both good and bad)
↓
Analyze, theorize and conclude the learning
↓
Action plan for future

REFLECTIVE WRITING

PORTFOLIO (PART A)

Name of Student: _____   Roll. No.: _____

Subject: _____   Batch: _____

Reflection on achievement of the competency (Number and Name):

_____
_____
_____
_____
_____

The reflection must be completed by the student immediately after completion of the competency.

_____
_____
_____
_____
_____

Self-reflection of the student (what happened, so what, what next)	Word Limit: 250

Competency-Based Logbook in Obstetrics and Gynecology for MBBS

My Three Most Important Learning Experiences in this Session

1.

2.

3.

Feedback from the Faculty

The following measures were agreed by student in order to achieve the competency:

_____
_____
_____
_____
_____
_____
_____
_____
_____
_____
_____
_____

Signature of Student   **Signature of Faculty**

List of Procedures and Surgeries Assisted/Observed

Sl. No.	Surgery observed/assisted	Date	Faculty feedback	Faculty signature

CERTIFIABLE COMPETENCY (AS PER CBME)

Sl. No.	Competencies	Number required to certify	Date of completion	Attestation by unit head (with date)	Attestation of department head
OG13.5	Observe and assist the conduct of a normal vaginal delivery.	10			

OTHER CERTIFIABLE COMPETENCIES

Sl. No.	Competencies	Number required to certify	Date of completion	Attestation by unit head (with date)	Attestation of department head
	IInd year				
OG35.1	Obtain a logical sequence of history and perform a humane and thorough clinical examination, excluding internal examination (per-rectal and per-vaginal).				
OG35.5	Determine gestational age, EDD and obstetric formula.				
OG8.3	Describe, demonstrate, document and perform an obstetrical examination including a general and abdominal examination and clinical monitoring of maternal and fetal well-being.	10			
OG8.5	Describe and demonstrate pelvic assessment in a model.	1			
	IIIrd year				
OG35.17	Demonstrate the correct technique of urinary catheterization in a simulated/supervised environment.				
	IVth year				
OG33.3	Describe and demonstrate the screening for cervical cancer in a simulated environment.				
OBG 15.2	• Observe and assist in the performance of an episiotomy in a simulated environment. • Observe/assist in operative cases including CS, forceps, vacuum extraction and breech delivery.				
OG35.15	Demonstrate the correct technique to insert and remove an IUD in a simulated/supervised environment.				
OG35.10	Write a proper referral note to secondary or tertiary centers or to other physicians with all necessary details.				
OG20.2	In a simulated environment administer informed consent to a person wishing to undergo medical termination of pregnancy (MTP).				
OG35.3	Recognize situations, which call for urgent or early treatment at secondary and tertiary centers and make a prompt referral of such patients after giving first aid or emergency treatment.				
OG35.4	Demonstrate interpersonal and communication skills befitting a physician in order to discuss illness and its outcome with patient and family.				
OG35.6	Demonstrate ethical behavior in all aspects of medical practice.				
OG35.7	Obtain informed consent for any examination/procedure.				
OG35.11	Demonstrate the correct use of appropriate universal precautions for self-protection against HIV and hepatitis and counsel patients.				

Sl. No.	Competencies	Number required to certify	Date of completion	Attestation by unit head (with date)	Attestation of department head
OB18.2	Demonstrate the steps of neonatal resuscitation in a simulated environment.				
OG17.2	Counsel in a simulated environment, care of the breast, importance and the technique of breastfeeding.				
OG9.2	Describe the steps and observe/assist in the performance of an MTP evacuation.				
OG13.3	Observe/assist in the performance of an artificial rupture of membranes.				
OG35.2	Arrive at a logical provisional diagnosis after examination.				
OG35.8	Write a complete case record with all necessary details.				
OG35.9	Write a proper discharge summary with all relevant information.				
OG35.12	Obtain a PAP smear in a simulated environment.				
OG19.2	Counsel in a stimulated environment, contraception and puerperal sterilization.				